About the author

Patrick Holford is one of the world's leading authorities on new approaches to health and nutrition. In 1984 he founded the Institute for Optimum Nutrition (ION), a charitable and independent educational trust for the furtherance of education and research in nutrition. Patrick Holford is one of Britain's leading spokespeople on nutrition and health issues and during the last decade has written 15 books, including the best-selling *The Optimum Nutrition Bible*.

What is optimum nutrition?

Optimum nutrition simply means giving your body the best possible intake of nutrients to allow it to be as healthy as possible and to work as well as it can.

Through optimum nutrition you can improve mental clarity and concentration, increase physical performance, boost your resistance to infections, protect yourself from disease and extend your healthy life span. By dipping into the advice in this book, you can add life to your years and years to your life.

*Let food be your medicine and
medicine be your food.*
Hippocrates, AD 390

Rise and shine

Encourage your body to
wake up in the mornings by having
a brief cold shower after
a hot shower.
This stimulates circulation
and digestion.

Wait for breakfast

Wait until you are totally awake
in the morning before eating –
your body won't be able to digest food
if it is still asleep.

Leave at least an hour between
waking up and breakfast, although if
you can't wait that long,
you can have a fresh fruit salad.

You'll function best on easy-to-digest
carbohydrate-based breakfasts
such as fruit or cereal,
rather than high-protein cooked
breakfasts.

Echinacea

A great all-rounder with anti-viral
and anti-bacterial properties.
The active ingredients
are thought to be
specific mucopolysaccharides.

Echinacea comes in capsules and
in extracts, taken as drops.

Don't get off to a bad start

Never start your day with
a stimulant (tea, coffee or a cigarette)
because the 'stress' state
these induce inhibits digestion.

Snack on fresh fruit

Eat 3 to 4 pieces of fresh fruit a day.

This will keep your
blood sugar levels even, giving you
more consistent energy,
moods and concentration.

Take regular exercise

Make sure you take some form
of exercise every day.
A sedentary lifestyle can lead to poor
appetite control and you will
eat more calories compared to their
expenditure than if you have
a more active lifestyle.

Maximise your fertility

For the best chance of a healthy baby,
both you and your partner
should prepare for pregnancy.
It takes 3 months for sperm
to mature, while the
egg or ovum takes a month.

During these pre-conceptual months
you should both pursue
optimum nutrition and minimise
your intake of anti-nutrients,
especially alcohol, as well as
abstaining from sex during
the non-fertile phases of the month.

Raw or cooked?

Eat as much raw or lightly cooked
food as you can.

Cooking changes the molecules
in food and destroys many
valuable nutrients and the enzymes
that break food down
into components that can be used
by the body.

The whole truth

Make sure you include plenty of whole foods in your diet:

- whole grains
- lentils
- beans
- nuts
- seeds
- fresh fruit and vegetables

There is no substitute for whole foods, which contain hundreds of health-promoting substances.

Should I supplement?

Even if you eat all the right foods,
you are unlikely to achieve
an optimal intake of all
the necessary vitamins and minerals.
Although everyone's
nutritional needs are different,
you should take a good multivitamin
and multimineral supplement
and additional vitamin C every day.

Is tap water fit to drink?

Drink bottled, distilled or filtered
water, not tap water, to
avoid pollutants but remember
that filtering and distilling water
removes not only impurities but also
many of the naturally occurring
minerals. This pushes up the need
for minerals from food.

Out of the frying pan

Grill, steam, boil or bake your food –
don't fry.

Frying food in oil produces
free radicals, highly reactive chemicals
that destroy essential fats
in food and can damage cells,
increasing the risk of cancer, heart
disease and premature ageing.

The fats of life

Many of us eat too much saturated fat,
the kind that kills, and too little of
the essential fats, the kind that heal.
Certain polyunsaturated fats, called
Omega 3 oils, found in pumpkin
and flax seeds and Omega 6 oils,
found in sesame and sunflower seeds,
are vital for our health.

To make sure you are getting enough,
eat 1 tablespoon of cold-pressed
seed oil (sesame, sunflower, pumpkin
or flax seed) or 1 heaped tablespoon
of ground seeds a day.

Fats that kill

Cut down on the fats that are bad
for you, found in meat and
dairy products — avoid
fried foods, burnt or browned fat,
saturated or hydrogenated fat.

Get enough protein

Eat 2 servings a day of

- beans
- lentils
- quinoa
- tofu (soya)
- 'seed' vegetables (such as peas, broad beans)
- *or* other vegetable protein
- *or* 1 small serving of meat, fish, cheese or a free-range egg.

Avoid too much meat and eat fish instead.

Slow, slow, quick, quick, slow

Carbohydrate is the body's
main fuel. It comes in two forms:

- 'fast-releasing' (as in sugar, honey, malt, sweets and most refined foods)
- 'slow-releasing' (as in whole grains, vegetables and fresh fruit).

The latter contain more complex carbohydrates and more fibre, both of which help to slow down the release of sugar. Fast-releasing carbohydrates are best avoided; slow-releasing ones should make up about two-thirds of your diet.

A regular dose of fibre

You should aim for a daily intake
of 35 grams of fibre. Fibre absorbs
water in the digestive tract,
making the food contents bulkier
and easier to pass through the body,
preventing constipation and
the putrefaction of foods.
This also slows down the absorption
of sugar into the blood, helping
to maintain good energy levels.

Top 5 diet tips

Your daily diet should include:

- 1 heaped tablespoon of ground seeds or 1 tablespoon of cold-pressed seed oil
- 3 servings beans, lentils, quinoa, tofu (soya) or 'seed' vegetables
- 3 pieces of fresh fruit such as apples, pears, berries, melon or citrus fruit
- 3 servings of dark green, leafy and root vegetables
- 4 servings of whole grains

Graze, don't gorge

Studies have shown that people
who eat little and often are
healthier than those who just eat
1 or 2 large meals a day.
In practice this means having breakfast,
lunch and dinner plus a couple
of snacks of fruit in between.

The healthy vegetarian

For a healthy vegetarian diet don't rely solely on cheese and eggs as sources of protein. Include plenty of beans, soya, lentils, seeds, nuts and whole grains, such as quinoa, millet and brown rice.

Breakfast like a king,
lunch like a prince,
dine like a pauper

There's a lot of truth to this old saying. You need food for energy during the day, so it doesn't make sense to eat half your day's food in the evening. Also, it's not a good idea to go to bed still digesting your supper. As a general rule, eat dinner early and leave at least 2 hours before going to bed.

Chew your food thoroughly

Chewing your food thoroughly
and eating at regular times
will help you to digest
and get the most out of your food.

Eat something raw
with every meal

The healthiest diet has
a large proportion of raw or
very lightly cooked food,
so serve something raw
with every meal.

The anti-stress diet

Fast-releasing sugars create a state
of stress in the body,
stimulating the release of cortisol.
So avoid eating white bread,
sweets and breakfast cereals or
other foods with added sugar.

Slow-releasing carbohydrates –
fruit, whole grains, beans, lentils,
nuts and seeds – on the other hand,
provide an 'even keel' of
consistent energy.

Increase your antioxidant levels

Boost your immune system and
improve your resistance to disease
by increasing your antioxidant levels.
Their presence in your diet and levels
in your blood may prove to be
the best marker yet of your power
to delay death and prevent disease.
The most important are:

- vitamin A – found in meat and fish
- vitamin C – abundant in
raw fruit and vegetables
- vitamin E – found in seed foods
- plus beta-carotene – found in red,
orange and yellow fruit and vegetables.

Sources of fibre

It is best to get fibre from a mixture of sources such as:

- oats
- lentils
- beans
- seeds
- fruits
- raw or lightly cooked vegetables

Much of the fibre in vegetables is destroyed by cooking, so they are best eaten crunchy.

Cat's claw

Cat's claw is a powerful anti-viral, antioxidant and immune-boosting agent from the Peruvian rainforest plant *Uncaria tomentosa*. It is available as a tea or in supplements.

Try cat's claw tea with added blackcurrant and apple concentrate; I cup a day helps maintain immune power. If you have a sore throat or stomach upset, add 4 slices of root ginger.

Water, water everywhere

The ideal daily water intake
is around 2 litres (3½ pints),
so make sure you are drinking enough.
4 pieces of fruit and 4 servings of
vegetables can provide about
a litre (1¾ pints) of water a day,
leaving a daily litre to be taken as
water or in the form of diluted
juices or herb and fruit teas.

Carbohydrates – the optimum daily intake

Eat:

- 3 or more servings of dark green, leafy and root vegetables, raw or lightly cooked
- 3 or more servings of fresh fruit
- 4 or more servings of whole grains

Avoid any form of sugar, foods with added sugar, white or refined foods.

Body robbers

Cut down on your intake of
alcohol, tea and coffee. These act as
diuretics, causing your body
to lose water as well as robbing it
of natural minerals.
Aim for no more than 1 unit of
alcohol a day (e.g. a glass of wine,
half a pint of beer or
lager or 1 measure of spirits).

Avoid hormone-disrupting chemicals

Minimise the amount of food,
especially wet or fatty food,
which you buy in direct contact
with soft plastic.
Hormone-disrupting chemicals
are used to soften plastic and can
end up in your food.
Glass bottles are better than
plastic bottles and paper bags are
better than plastic ones.
Hard plastic is less likely
to be a problem.

Maintain a balance

Do not supplement your diet with
individual nutrients without also
taking a good all-round multivitamin
and mineral supplement.

Mind your minerals

Eat 1 serving of mineral-rich foods
such as kale, cabbage,
root vegetables, low-fat dairy products
such as yoghurt, seeds or nuts
such as almonds, as well as plenty
of fresh fruit, vegetables and
whole foods such as lentils, beans
and whole grains every day.

From small seeds

All 'seed' foods, which include

- seeds
- nuts
- lentils
- dried beans
- peas
- broad beans
- runner beans
- whole grains

– are good sources of iron, zinc, manganese and chromium. Make sure you get plenty in your diet.

Green foods

Green foods are a rich source of
chlorophyll and magnesium
which is vital for the nerves, muscles
and balancing hormones.

Pure, organic food

Choose organic foods whenever possible
to try and eat as near as you can get
to a pure diet and to avoid
possible contamination with hormones
and antibiotics.

Gluten free

If you have gluten sensitivity,
try rice, corn, quinoa and buckwheat
which are all gluten free.

Vitamin C

As well as a high-strength
multivitamin and mineral preparation,
take 1000mg of vitamin C
every day.

Just say no

Avoid any form of sugar,
also white, refined or processed food
with chemical additives,
and minimise your intake of alcohol,
coffee or tea.

The key to good health

Improving your digestion is the
cornerstone to good health.
Energy levels improve, the skin
becomes softer and clearer,
body odour reduces and the
immune system is strengthened.

The trick is to work from the top down,
first ensuring good digestion,
then good absorption and finally
good elimination.

Soya – a top protein food

Soya is a prime source of good protein so try and include it in your diet.

The easiest way to eat soya is in the form of tofu, a curd made from beans. There are many kinds of tofu – soft, hard, marinated, smoked, braised. Soft tofu can be used to give a creamy texture to soups and hard tofu can be cubed and used in vegetable stir-fries, stews and casseroles.

Is meat healthy?

It is good health advice to reduce
your consumption of meat,
especially the types that contain
high levels of saturated fat,
and eat vegetable foods (beans,
lentils or whole grains),
free-range chicken or fish instead.

Frequent shopper

Buy fresh foods little and often.
Keeping them
destroys their nutrients.

A seedy mix

Put I measure each of sesame,
sunflower and pumpkin seeds
and 2 measures of flax seeds in
a sealed jar and keep it in the fridge,
away from light, heat and air.
Grinding 2 tablespoons of these seeds
in a coffee grinder and
adding them to your daily breakfast
cereal will guarantee a
good intake of essential fatty acids.

Warning – frying can seriously damage your health

Frying damages healthy oils.
The high temperature makes the oil
oxidise which generates
harmful free radicals. Frying is
therefore best avoided but
if you do fry, use a tiny amount of
olive oil or butter because they are
less prone to oxidation than top-quality
cold-pressed vegetable oils.

Balance your blood sugar

Keeping your blood sugar balanced
is probably the most important
factor in maintaining even energy
levels and weight.
An estimated 3 in 10 of us have
impaired ability to keep our
blood sugar level even and the result,
over the years, is that we become
increasingly fat and lethargic.
But if you can control your
blood sugar levels the result is even
weight and constant energy.

Grapefruit seed extract

If you have a bacterial, fungal or parasitical infection take 10 drops of grapefruit seed extract 2 or 3 times a day. It has a similar effect to antibiotics but doesn't damage beneficial gut bacteria as conventional antibiotics do.

Cut down on sugar

Reduce the sugar content of
your diet by gradually getting used
to less sweetness.

Try sweetening breakfast cereal
with fruit, dilute fruit juices
50:50 with water,
limit your intake of dried fruit and
avoid foods with added sugar.

Double or quit

If you smoke, drink alcohol, live in a
polluted city, are pre-menstrual,
menopausal, on the pill, exercise a lot, are
fighting an infection or stressed out,
your nutrient needs can easily double.
Make sure you are getting enough.

Quality, not quantity

While it's great to eat lots of fruit
and vegetables, the quality
is just as important as the quantity.
For this reason, it's best to
buy local produce in season and
consume it quickly.
The worst thing you can do is buy
fruit shipped in from the other side
of the world, and leave it hanging around
for 2 weeks before you eat it.

Magnesium

A lack of magnesium is
strongly associated with
cardiovascular disease so eat plenty
of green vegetables, nuts
and seeds to avoid deficiency.

Blue and purple foods

Beetroot, red grapes and berries
derive their red, blue and purple hues
from a group of
phytonutrients called flavonoids.
These are very powerful antioxidants.
The protective effect of red wine
on cardiovascular disease
is probably due to these.

Among the most powerful
flavonoids are anthocyanidins
which give the purple colour to
blueberries, blackberries,
blackcurrant and red grapes.

Quinoa – a near perfect food

Experiment with quinoa.
Called the mother grain because of
its sustaining properties, quinoa
contains protein of a better quality
than that of meat. Although known
as a grain, it's technically a fruit.
Nutritionally it is quite unique,
containing more protein than a grain
and more essential fat than
fruit. It is also rich in vitamins and
minerals and it's about as close
to a perfect food as you can get.
It cooks in 15 minutes, like rice.

Selenium – the anti-cancer mineral

Selenium has protective properties against cancer and premature ageing.
It is found predominantly in whole foods, particularly nuts, seafood, seaweed and sesame seeds.
Grind the seeds to make the nutrients more readily available.

Top foods for boosting your antioxidant levels

Eating sweet potatoes, carrots, watercress, peas and broccoli frequently is a great way to increase your antioxidant potential – provided, of course, that you don't fry them.

Watermelons

Eat watermelons.

The flesh is high in beta-carotene
and vitamin C, while
the seeds are high in vitamin E
and in the antioxidant minerals
zinc and selenium.

Blend the seeds and flesh
in a blender for a pollution-busting
antioxidant cocktail.

The protectors

Eat more white meat, tuna,
lentils, beans, nuts, seeds, onions
and garlic.

They are high in the amino acids
cysteine and glutathione
which act as antioxidants.

They enable you to make an enzyme
which helps detoxify the body,
protecting you against car fumes,
carcinogens, infections, excess
alcohol and toxic metals.

Build the blood

Eat plenty of chlorophyll-rich
foods such as wheat grass, algae,
seaweeds and green vegetables
to help 'build' your blood.

Vitamins C, B2, B6, A, K
and folic acid are
among the nutrients needed
to keep the blood healthy.

A tomato a day

Include plenty of tomatoes,
green peppers, pineapples,
strawberries and carrots in your diet.

These have high levels of
coumarins and chlorogenic acid
which prevent the formation of
cancer-causing nitrosamines.

Berry good

Tuck into strawberries, raspberries
or a bunch of grapes.

All these are high in ellagic acid
which neutralises carcinogens before
they can damage your DNA.

Enzymes – the key to life

The food you eat cannot
nourish you unless it is first prepared
for absorption into the body.
This is done by enzymes,
chemical compounds that digest
it and break down large
food particles into smaller units.

A good way of boosting your
enzyme potential is to eat raw foods,
because in this state they
contain significant amounts
of enzymes. The cooking process
tends to destroy them.

Supplement your antioxidants

Take a comprehensive antioxidant supplement, especially if you are middle-aged or older, live in a polluted city or suffer any other unavoidable exposure to free radicals.

Bioflavonoids

Boost your bioflavonoid levels.
Bioflavonoids are potent antioxidants which
can bind to toxic metals and escort them
out of the body; they have a synergistic
effect on vitamin C, stabilising it in human
tissue; they have an antibiotic effect and
they are also anti-carcinogenic.
Best food sources are:

- berries
- buckwheat leaves
- tea
- citrus fruit

- grapes
- papaya
- broccoli
- plums
- red wine

- rosehips
- cherries
- tomatoes
- cantaloupe melons

Improve your memory and mental performance

Reduce your intake of stimulants, sugar and refined foods; minimise your exposure to pollution and cigarettes; make sure you are 'well oiled' with regular seeds, their oils or essential fat supplements, and take a high-dose multivitamin and mineral supplement.

Bring colour into your life

Eat something green, yellow, orange, red and blue every day – each natural colour contains different health-promoting phytochemicals.

Buying, storing and preparing food

The 3 main enemies of vitamins
and minerals are heating,
water and oxidation so:

- eat foods as fresh and unprocessed
  as possible
- keep fresh food cool and in the dark
  in the fridge in sealed containers
- eat more raw food
- cook foods as whole as possible
- steam or boil foods with as
  little water as possible
- avoid frying food.

Maximum immunity

For maximum immunity, eat a
well-balanced protein, low-fat diet,
with fats obtained from
essential sources such as seeds and nuts,
together with plenty of fresh fruit
and vegetables rich
in vitamins and minerals.

Improve your digestion

Eating 80 per cent alkaline-forming
foods and 20 per cent
acid-forming foods will help
improve your digestion.
This means eating large quantities
of vegetables and fruit, and
less concentrated protein foods like
beans, lentils and whole grains
instead of meat, fish, cheese and eggs.

To combine, or not to combine?

Eat animal protein on its own or
with vegetables. Concentrated protein
like meat, fish, hard cheese
and eggs require lots of stomach acid
and a stay of about 3 hours
in the stomach to be digested.
So do not combine fast-releasing
or refined carbohydrates or food that
ferments with animal protein.

Avoid acid stomach

If you suffer from 'acid stomach',
experienced as indigestion and a burning
sensation, avoid acid-forming and
irritating foods and drinks; alcohol, coffee,
tea and aspirin all irritate the gut wall.
Meat, fish and other proteins
stimulate acid production and can
aggravate over-acidity.

Constipation – natural solutions

Make sure you eat plenty of fruit,
vegetables and whole grains,
plus drink lots of water.
Exercise that stimulates the abdominal
area also helps to improve
digestion, as do breathing exercises
that relax the abdomen.
It is a natural reflex of the body
to stop digesting in times of stress.

Lower your blood pressure

Your arteries are surrounded by
a layer of muscle and an excess of
sodium, or a lack of calcium,
magnesium or potassium,
can increase the muscular pressure.
Increasing your intake of
these minerals, while avoiding
added salt (sodium chloride),
can make a substantial difference to
your blood pressure in a month.
Solo salt, rich in magnesium,
is a healthy substitute.

The right sort of exercise

Take up tai-chi.

While over-training or vigorous exercise can actually suppress the immune system, the gentle Chinese art of tai-chi has been shown to increase the count of T-cells (one of the body's types of immune cells) by 40 per cent.

Top of the immune-boosting nutrients

Vitamin C is unquestionably the master immune-boosting nutrient.

It helps immune cells to mature, improves the performance of antibodies and macrophages and is itself anti-viral and anti-bacterial, as well as being able to destroy toxins produced by bacteria. It's also a natural anti-histamine, calming down inflammation.

Salad days

To boost your immune system
combine the following in a large salad:

- a selection of 'seed' vegetables
- broccoli
- grated carrot
- beetroot
- courgettes
- watercress
- lettuce
- tomatoes
- avocados

and add seeds or marinated tofu
pieces. Serve with a dressing
of cold-pressed oil containing
some crushed garlic.

Stress and the adrenals

If you live off stimulants such as
coffee and cigarettes,
high-sugar diets or stress itself
you increase your risk of upsetting
your thyroid balance (which
means your metabolism will
slow down and you will gain weight),
your calcium balance (resulting in
arthritis), or of getting problems
associated with sex-hormone
imbalances. Make those all-important
lifestyle changes.

Yellow foods

Yellow foods, such as
sweetcorn and yellow peppers,
are rich in carotenoids,
powerful antioxidants that protect
you from cancer.

Mustard and the spice turmeric,
the main ingredients in curry powder,
are both rich in the
pigment curcumin. This is a powerful
phytonutrient known to fight cancer
and to reduce inflammation
suffered by people with arthritis.

Reduce your risk of osteoporosis

Some medical scientists now believe that a life-long consumption of a high-protein, acid-forming diet may be a primary cause of osteoporosis, so reducing your meat consumption is a sensible precaution.

Time for fruit

The best time to eat fruit
is as a snack more than 30 minutes
before a meal,
or not less than 2 hours
after a meal.

What you eat today, you wear tomorrow

Nutrition is fundamentally
involved at every stage
of skin development.

Limit damage caused by
free radicals by ensuring a diet
rich in antioxidants such as
vitamins A, C and E, and selenium.

Combating skin problems

If you have skin problems,
limit alcohol, coffee, tea, sugar
and saturated fat
(as in meat and dairy products)
and increase your intake of
fresh fruit, vegetables, water,
herb teas and diluted juices.

Also take a good
all-round multivitamin and mineral
supplement, plus at least
1000mg of vitamin C a day.

Fish with bite

Eat 3 servings of fish a week,
especially if this is your only source
of essential fats.

The best fish to eat are fish with teeth,
such as herring, mackerel,
tuna or salmon which are especially
rich in the most powerful of all
Omega 3 oils, known as DHA
and EPA. Having a good intake of
these is linked with better
brain function and memory, and less
risk of cancer and heart disease.

Cellulite

Apples are particularly good
at eliminating cellulite.

The pectin found in apples,
carrots and other fruit and
vegetables is an important
phytochemical which strengthens
the immune and detoxification
systems of the body.

Consider a 3-day apple fast or eat only
organic apples 1 day a week.

The brain drain

While so called 'good' chemicals and nutrients can improve mental function, 'bad' chemicals can and do reduce your intelligence. Alcohol is a prime example. Coffee, while commonly thought to improve concentration, actually diminishes it. Boost your energy with a fruit snack instead.

The energy equation

To maximise your available energy for life,
and to retain that energy rather than
burning out, eat slow-releasing
carbohydrates that release their 'fuel'
slowly, ensure you have optimal intakes
of all essential nutrients,
and avoid stimulants and depressants.

The breath of life

Deeper breathing not only energises the body, it also clears the mind.

Mastering the right way to breathe is the first step in most forms of meditation, yoga and tai-chi so why not join a class and reap the benefits?

Psychocalisthenics

Try an exercise system called
Psychocalisthenics.

It's a unique series of 22 exercises which
develop strength, suppleness and stamina
and oxygenate the whole body.

Find a class and join in.
It's easy to learn in a day and suitable
for young and old alike.

Lean cuisine

The leaner you are, the longer you are likely to live. Many foods in today's diet provide 'empty' calories – sugar or saturated fat, but none of the micronutrients needed to process them. These foods are out if you want to extend your life span.

Nutrient-dense foods such as organic carrots, apples, nuts and seeds provide as many nutrients as calories plus, in the case of fresh fruit and vegetables, plenty of essential and calorie-free water.

Restrict your calories

One way to restrict calories
is simply to eat less. Another is to fast
or have a modified fast 1 day
a week. This may mean, for example,
eating only fruit. Keep your overall
intake low by eating a substantial
breakfast and dinner but a small lunch
(or no lunch at all but snacks
of fruit throughout the day).

Maximise your healthy life span

Stay away from avoidable sources
of free radicals, for example fried
or browned foods, exhaust fumes,
smoke and strong sunlight.

Defeat arthritis

Cut down on refined sugar, stimulants, saturated fat and protein. Too much of all of these is strongly associated with arthritic problems.

The healthy vegan

For a healthy vegan diet include plenty of beans, soya, lentils, seeds and nuts. Also include whole grains, such as quinoa, millet and brown rice.

Take a good multivitamin and multimineral supplement which includes vitamins D and B12.

Cancer-fighting foods

Eating certain kinds of food is associated with a decreased risk of cancer. Try adding the following foods to your diet:

- fruit and vegetables, especially ones containing beta-carotene such as carrots, broccoli, sweet potatoes, cantaloupe melons and apricots
- garlic
- soya beans
- live yoghurt
- sesame and sunflower seeds

Eat lightly when you're ill

If you are suffering from an infection,
it is best to eat lightly – small meals
made from high-energy natural foods,
raw or lightly cooked.

During an infection the body fights
hard to eliminate the waste products
of war, so drink plenty of water
or herb tea to help your body
detoxify and reduce mucus.

How to kill a cold

While a gram of vitamin C a day
helps to reduce the severity
and incidence of colds,
achieving 'tissue saturation' has even
greater results. To get to this point, take in
around 10-15 grams a day,
or 3 grams every 4 hours,
which is 375 times the RDA.

Increase your energy

To experience substantially more
energy and ability to cope
with stress, cut out stimulants and
start taking nutritional support.

Coffee, tea and chocolate are best
omitted altogether –
decaffeinated coffee and tea
still contain stimulants.

There are plenty of coffee alternatives
and herb and fruit teas.
Healthfood shops also have
sugar-free 'sweets' and bars but check
the label for hidden sugar.

Immune~boosting herbs

Stock up on immune-boosting herbs
which help fight infection.
These are excellent:

- cat's claw
- echinacea
- garlic
- grapefruit seed extract

Ginger

Ginger is good for sore throats and stomach upsets.

Put 6 slices of fresh root ginger in a thermos with a stick of cinnamon and fill it up with boiling water. Five minutes later you have a delicious, throat-soothing tea. Add a little lemon or honey to taste.

The magic of mushrooms

Shiitake, maiitake, reishi, ganoderma
and other mushrooms have been
shown to be immune-boosting.
You can find them added to some
immune-boosting supplements and tonics
or you can buy shiitake fresh
in the supermarket or dried in
healthfood shops.

Take up meditation

For maximum energy, eat pure food
and have pure thoughts.
Meditation is as important to
the mind as food is to the body.
It's a time you set aside to sit
in silence, focusing on something
simple like the breath or a prayer,
and letting go of your endless
stream of thoughts and tapping
into the source of energy
within every human being,
from which comes creativity, joy,
natural humour and lightness.

Your weight is a burning issue

Get your metabolism working for you rather than against you. A crash diet of below 1000 calories a day will merely cause your body to feel under threat and it slows down the metabolic rate by as much as 45 per cent. It's not just how much food that makes a difference, but the kind of food you eat. Eat slow-releasing carbohydrates which produce a more consistent energy level, longer relief from hunger and give your body a better chance to use up the food rather than turning it to fat.

Watermelon cocktail

Blend the flesh and seeds of a watermelon in an electric blender. The husks will sink to the bottom, leaving the seeds, which are rich in protein, zinc, selenium, vitamin E and essential fats, in the juice.

To detox drink a pint for breakfast and another pint during the day.

Mums-to-be

If you are pregnant, your need for
vitamins B6 and B12, folic acid,
iron and zinc all increase.
Supplementing these usually stops
even the worst cases of
morning sickness.

Keeping food fresh

Keep fresh food in the fridge
in sealed containers –
cool, covered and in the dark.

Elderberry extract

If you have a cold,
take 1 teaspoon of Sambucol
(elderberry extract)
4 times a day.

Vary your diet

Eat a varied diet,
choosing from the widest possible
range of foods.

Hidden sugars

Very few breakfast cereals are truly
sugar-free: most processed cereals
contain fast-releasing sugars and
have added sugar.

Try oats, sugar-free cornflakes
or millet flakes instead and
sweeten the cereal with fruit
such as a sliced banana, apple or pear.

Fruit, not sweets

Always have a fruit bowl packed with fresh, appealing fruit to snack on during the day. Send kids to school with fruit rather than money to buy sweets.

Golden rules for a healthy diet

- Avoid sugar
- Avoid refined carbohydrates
- Eat more beans, lentils and whole grains
- Eat more vegetables, raw or lightly cooked
- Eat 3 pieces of fresh fruit a day
- Avoid coffee, tea and cigarettes
- Limit alcohol

Take your supplements regularly

Always take your supplements – irregular supplementation doesn't work. Vitamins and minerals are not drugs, so you should not expect an overnight improvement in your health.

Most people experience a definite improvement to their health within 3 months – the shortest length of time that you should experiment with a supplementation programme.

Not to be sneezed at

Take a daily supplement
of 1 gram of vitamin C or more
to reduce the incidence,
severity and duration of colds.

PMS sufferers

If you suffer from PMS, try eating little and often prior to menstruation, snacking on fruit but avoiding sugar, sweets and stimulants.

Ensure that your daily diet contains 1 tablespoon of cold-pressed vegetable oil rich in both Omega 3 and Omega 6 fatty acids.

Feed your brain

If you want your brain to be in peak condition, eat plenty of sardines. These are a good source of brain nutrients.

Trouble sleeping?

If you have problems sleeping,
avoid all stimulants.

Do not eat sugar or drink tea or coffee in
the evening and don't eat late at night.

Eat seeds, nuts, root and green leafy
vegetables which are high in calcium
and magnesium (which have a
tranquillising effect).

Water with wine

Alcohol is a diuretic so it dehydrates you. The healthiest recommendation is not to drink at all, or to limit your intake to 3 or 4 drinks a week (preferably of red wine). When drinking alcohol, drink some water with it to prevent dehydration.

Fat intake

Of your total fat intake, no more
than one-third should be
saturated (hard) fat, and at least
one-third should be polyunsaturated oils,
with the remaining third coming from
monounsaturated fat. To achieve this,
eat less meat and dairy produce, and
more fish, seeds and their oils.

Try an oil blend

Some companies produce special cold-pressed oil blends containing different proportions of flax seed oil and other oils to give you the right balance of Omega 3 and Omega 6 oils. These oil blends, or flax seed oil, are the best to use, but don't fry with them and keep them in the fridge.

Dry skin

Drink at least 1 litre (1¾ pints)
of water a day and eat plenty of
water-rich foods such as fruit
and vegetables. Alcohol, tea and coffee
should be limited. Make sure
your diet is low in saturated fat
and high in essential fatty oils
(from seeds and their oils).

Cut out margarine

Cut out margarine and try tahini (sesame spread) or olive oil instead.

The refining and processing of vegetable oils during the manufacture of margarine can change the nature of the polyunsaturated oil. To turn the oil into a hard fat it is 'hydrogenated' and the body cannot make use of it. Even worse it blocks the body's ability to use healthy polyunsaturated oils.

Reverse the ageing process

Slow down the ageing process by
decreasing your exposure to oxidants,
increasing your intake of antioxidant
nutrients from diet and supplements,
and eating less quantity and more
quality foods.

Limit your exposure to oxidants

By limiting your exposure to burnt, browned or fried foods, you limit your exposure to oxidants. Try other cooking methods such as steam-frying, poaching, boiling and baking.

Eat your greens

Cruciferous vegetables (whose leaves grow in a cross pattern) are especially rich in certain phytonutrients. These are powerful detoxifying substances and can help break down cancer-causing chemicals. Eat:

- broccoli
- Brussels sprouts
- cabbage
- cauliflower
- cress
- horseradish
- kale
- kohlrabi
- mustard relish
- turnip

If you eat cabbage more than once a week, research shows you are only one-third as likely to develop cancer as someone who never eats cabbage.

Top infection-fighting foods

If you're fighting an infection,
the best vitamin C-rich
foods for the job are
blueberries or blackcurrants.

A traveller's tip

As garlic gives viruses, bacteria and parasites a hard time, it's a great food to include in your daily diet when travelling in parts of the world where the risk of picking up a stomach bug is high. Ideally, you should have 1 or 2 cloves a day.

Healthy bacteria

Promoting healthy bacteria
is an important part of keeping
your body free from infection.
And this is where fermented foods,
such as yoghurt, can help.
Only buy live yoghurt.

Salt substitute

Don't add salt to your food when cooking and reduce your consumption of foods with added salt.

Icelandic salt, marketed as Solo salt, is a healthy alternative to regular salt. It has more or less equal proportions of sodium and potassium, plus significant quantities of magnesium.

Reduce the risk of heart disease

Eating fish 3 times a week,
especially if this is instead of meat,
is a key factor in reducing
your risk of heart disease
in later life.

For vegetarians,
the best alternative sources
of Omega 3 fats are
flax seeds and their oil.

Wholefoods

Eat wholefoods as much as possible.

That means brown rice, brown bread, wholewheat pasta and naturally wholefoods such as nuts, seeds, lentils, beans, vegetables and fruit.

The cutting edge

To preserve their nutrient content,
cut up fresh foods just before
you are about to use them.
As soon as a large amount of the
surface area inside a plant
is exposed to oxygen, nutrient losses
are rapid.

Steam-frying

Use steam-frying as an alternative to frying. This involves frying foods with a very small amount of oil and some water, vegetable stock, soya sauce or some other water-based sauce. As soon as the lid is put on, the foods are effectively steamed.

Feeding your baby

Healthy babies, like healthy adults,
need food that is fresh, unprocessed,
additive-free, sugar-free, salt-free and low
in fat. In other words you should give
your baby food that is close to how
it is found in nature.

A hearty appetite

If you eat the right things,
heart disease is preventable.

Key prevention foods are fruit and
vegetables that are rich in
antioxidants such as beta-carotene
and vitamin C; fish and seeds,
rich in vitamin E and essential fats;
and garlic.

It's also important to cut down on
sugar, saturated fat and salt.

Fighting viral infection

At the first sign of a viral infection
(e.g. cold or flu):

- increase your vitamin C intake
to 3000mg every 4 hours;
- suck zinc lozenges;
- drink 2 cups of cat's claw tea a day
(made from the loose herb
brewed in water, not teabags);
- and take 4 dessertspoons of
black elderberry extract (Sambucol)
a day.

The travel bug

If on holiday in a place where
you know hygiene standards are likely
to be low, take a
probiotic supplement such as
Lactobacillus acidophilus and
bifidus daily to build up
your beneficial bacteria. Also carry
grapefruit seed extract with you
and take 10 drops 2 or 3 times a day
if you suspect an infection.

Limit your exposure to pesticides

Eat organic food.
This instantly minimises your
exposure to pesticides
and herbicides.

When you are eating non-organic
produce, add 2 tablespoons of vinegar
to your bowl of washing water.
This will reduce pesticides.

Less animal fat

Reduce your intake of fatty foods.
Non-biodegradable chemicals
accumulate in the food chain in
animal fat. Minimising your intake
of animal fat – meat and
dairy produce – lessens your exposure.
There is no need to limit
essential fats in nuts and seeds.

Boosting the immune system

Keeping your body topped up
with enough vitamin C, E and
selenium will not only
make it difficult for a virus
to survive, but renders it
much less harmful.

Four steps to prolongevity

- Minimise your exposure to free radicals
- Choose food rich in antioxidants
- Supplement antioxidants
- Cut down on calories – try fasting or have a modified fast 1 day a week.

Orange and red foods

Orange and red foods often derive their colour from carotenoids such as beta-carotene. Tomatoes and watermelon are rich in another carotenoid called lycopene. These carotenoids are strong antioxidants and help keep you young and healthy. Best sources are food such as:

- apricots
- carrots
- mango
- melons
- papaya
- peaches
- tomatoes
- watermelon

Aloe vera

Try aloe vera as a good
all-round tonic, as well as a booster
during any infection.
It has immune boosting, anti-viral
and antiseptic properties.

Avoiding toxic elements

Try not to buy unwrapped fruit
and vegetables that do not
require peeling that have been
exposed to street traffic.

Zinc

Zinc is essential for both men
and women for fertility.
Tuck into some oysters – not only
an aphrodisiac but also the
highest dietary source of zinc.
Avoid stress, smoking and alcohol
which will all deplete
your natural store.

The four seasons

Choose fruit and vegetables
in season.

This means that your exposure
to the chemicals used to
delay ripening, prolong shelf-life,
preserve colour and so on
will be limited.

Relax

Practise relaxation or
meditation techniques that involve
deep breathing.

This helps to bring oxygen
to your cells and to combat the effects
of free radicals.

Painkillers

If you take painkillers regularly,
increase your daily vitamin C intake
by 1000mg.

Antibiotics

If you are on a course of antibiotics,
take a high-strength B complex
during the course,
and supplement beneficial bacteria
(such as *acidophilus*)
for 2 weeks after the course.

On the pill

If you are on the birth control pill,
take a high-strength B complex
and extra B6 (100mg a day)
plus 15mg zinc a day.

For the allergic

If you are allergic or chemically sensitive, you will notice a dramatic improvement if you change to drinking spring or properly filtered water instead of tap water.

Garlic

Garlic contains allicin which is
anti-viral, anti-fungal and anti-bacterial.
It also acts as an antioxidant,
being rich in sulphur-containing
amino acids.

It will help you fight infections
and is a wise addition to your diet
as garlic eaters have the lowest
reported incidence of cancer.

Consider a clove or
capsule equivalent for an easy guide
to your daily dose.

Pick or pull

Pure, unadulterated food is
what your body needs.
For optimum nutrition, try to ensure
that your diet consists of whole,
natural food that you could pick
from a tree, or pull from the ground,
free from pesticides, artificial
additives or genetic modification.

Diet for the 21st century

- Eat foods raw or lightly cooked
  - Add colour to your diet
  - Choose natural, organic
    and whole foods
- Bake, boil, steam or steam-fry,
  instead of oil-frying

Investment for the future

Invest in a professional
assessment of your nutrition needs
from a qualified
nutrition consultant.

Other books by Patrick Holford also published by Piatkus

The Optimum Nutrition Bible
100% Health
The Optimum Nutrition Cookbook (with Judy Ridgway)
6 Weeks to Superhealth
The 30-day Fatburner Diet
Balancing Hormones Naturally (with Kate Neil)
Beat Stress and Fatigue
Boost Your Immune System (with Jennifer Meek)
Improve Your Digestion
Say No to Arthritis
Say No to Cancer
Say No to Heart Disease
Supplements for Superhealth

Information on Optimum Nutrition

Visit www.patrickholford.com
for

- Your questions answered
- Referral to a nutritionist in your area
- To work out your vitamin needs
- A diary of courses and lectures
- Details on Patrick Holford's 100% Health newsletter
- and more

For a free information pack, write to:
The Institute for Optimum Nutrition,
Blades Court, Deodar Road,
London SW15 2NU.
Tel: 020 8877 9993. Fax: 020 8877 9980.